Table of Contents

PREVIEW

Myalgic encephalomyelitis/chronic fatigue syndrome (ME/CFS) is a complex and disabling disease. It has been classified as a neurological disorder by the World Health Organization, though it affects many parts of the body, including the brain and muscles, digestive, immune and cardiac systems.

The term 'myalgic encephalomyelitis' means pain in the muscles, and inflammation in the brain and spinal cord. Scientists are starting to understand some of the biological changes in the bodies of people with ME/CFS, although they have not yet found how to prevent, or cure it.

Research has found that ME/CFS is associated with problems involving:

The body's ability to produce energy at a cellular level

Immune, neurological and hormonal systems

Blood pressure and heart rate regulation

Digestion

Sleep

Cognition – how quickly information is processed

ME/CFS affects men, women and children of all ages, ethnicities, and socioeconomic backgrounds. 75-80% of people with the disease are female. It is estimated that up to 600,000 Victorians may be living with ME/CFS, and as many as 90% are undiagnosed.

The main symptom of ME/CFS is extreme physical and mental tiredness (fatigue) that does not go away with rest or sleep. This can make it difficult to carry out everyday tasks and activities.

Most people with ME/CFS describe their fatigue as overwhelming and a different type of tiredness from what they've experienced before.

Exercising usually makes the symptoms worse. Sometimes the effect is delayed and you'll feel very tired a few hours after you've exercised, or even the next day.

Symptoms vary from person to person, and the severity of symptoms can vary from day to day, or even within a day.

CHRONIC FATIGUE DIET RECIPES

BREAKFAST

1. Enchiladas

Prep Time: 25 Minutes

Cook Time: 20 Minutes

Servings: 8

Ingredients

- 2 (10 ounce) cans Old El Paso green enchilada sauce
- 1 tablespoon oil
- 12 ounces (about 14 links) breakfast sausage
- 12 eggs, whisked
- 8 Old El Paso large flour tortillas
- 1 (14-ounce) can black beans, rinsed and drained
- 2 avocados, peeled, pitted and diced
- 3 cups shredded Monterrey Jack or Pepper Jack cheese
- ½ cup chopped fresh cilantro leaves
- ¼ cup thinly-sliced green onions

Instructions

1. Preheat oven to 350 degrees F. Spray a large 9×13-inch baking dish with cooking spray. Then spread ⅓ cup Green Enchilada Sauce evenly along the bottom of the dish. Set aside.

2. Heat oil in a large saute pan over medium-high heat. Add sausage links (whole) and fry for 8-10 minutes, turning frequently, until golden brown. Transfer links to a separate plate, and reduce heat to medium-low. Add the eggs and cook for about 5-7 minutes until scrambled, stirring occasionally. Transfer eggs to a separate plate, and remove pan from heat. Cut the sausage links into small bite-sized pieces.

3. Set aside 1 cup of the shredded cheese, 1 avocado and 1/4 cup black beans for later use.

4. Lay a flour tortilla out a workspace. Spread 2 tablespoons green enchilada sauce all over the surface of the tortilla. Then in a line down the center, layer a large spoonful each of the eggs, sausage, avocado, cheese and beans. (Portion each ingredient so that you use about ⅛ of the entire portion per enchilada, since there are 8 total.) Fold the tortilla over to seal it, then transfer the enchilada to the pan. Repeat with the remaining tortillas until all 8 enchiladas are in the pan.

You may need to squish them together a bit to make room.

5. Spread about 1/2 cup of the remaining green enchilada sauce on top of the enchiladas. Then sprinkle the reserved 1 cup shredded cheese evenly on top. Bake for 20 minutes.

6. Remove, and sprinkle the enchiladas evenly with the reserved avocado, fresh cilantro, black beans and green onions, or whatever toppings you desire.

2. Easy Casserole with Sausage, Hashbrowns and Eggs

Prep Time: 15 Minutes

Cook Time: 30 Minutes

Servings: 8

Ingredients

- 1 pound ground Italian sausage (hot, mild or sweet)
- 1 medium white onion, diced
- 1 red bell pepper, cored and diced
- 3 cloves garlic, minced
- 1 (20 ounce) bag frozen diced hash brown potatoes,thawed
- 2 cups shredded sharp cheddar cheese, divided
- 6 eggs
- 1/3 cup milk
- 1 teaspoon fine sea salt
- A few generous twists of freshly-cracked black pepper
- Toppings: thinly sliced green onions, sliced avocado and/or hot sauce

Instructions

1. Prepare oven. Heat oven to 375°F.

2. Brown the sausage. Cook over medium-high heat in a large sauté pan until browned, crumbling the sausage with a spoon as it cooks. Transfer sausage with a slotted spoon to a large mixing bowl. Reserve 1 tablespoon of the remaining sausage grease in the sauté, and discard the rest.

3. Sauté veggies. Add onion and bell pepper to the pan and sauté for 5 minutes, stirring occasionally, until softened. Add garlic and sauté for an additional 2 minutes, stirring frequently, until fragrant. Transfer the vegetable mixture into the mixing bowl with the sausage. Add the thawed diced potatoes and 1 1/2 cups cheese to the mixing bowl with the sausage and veggies. Toss gently until evenly combined.

4. Add the eggs. In a separate small bowl, whisk together the eggs, milk, salt and black pepper until combined. Add the egg mixture to the potato mixture and toss gently to combine.

5. Bake. Pour the mixture into a 9×13-inch baking dish and top with the remaining 1/2 cup of shredded cheese. Cover with aluminum foil and bake for 40 minutes. Remove the aluminum foil and bake for an additional

10-15 minutes until the potatoes in the center are cooked through. Transfer the baking dish to a wire rack.

6. Serve. Serve warm, garnished with your favorite toppings, and enjoy!

3. Hummus and Veggies Bowl

Prep Time: 25 Minutes

Cook Time: 5 Minutes

Servings: 4

Ingredients

Breakfast Bowls Ingredients:

- 1 tablespoon avocado oil or olive oil
- 1 pound asparagus[1], cut into bite-sized pieces (with ends trimmed and discarded)
- 3 cups shredded kale leaves
- 1 batch lemony dressing
- 3 cups shredded (uncooked) Brussels sprouts[2]
- 1 ½ cups cooked quinoa[3]
- ½ cup hummus
- 1 avocado, peeled, pitted and thinly-sliced
- 4 eggs, cooked however you'd like (I soft-boiled mine)
- Garnishes: sunflower seeds (or sliced almonds), toasted sesame seeds, crushed red pepper

Lemony Dressing Ingredients:

- 2 tablespoons avocado oil or olive oil

- 2 tablespoons freshly-squeezed lemon juice
- 2 teaspoons Dijon mustard
- 1 garlic clove, minced
- Salt and freshly-cracked black pepper

Instructions

To Make The Breakfast Bowls:

1. Heat oil in a large saute pan over medium-high heat. Add asparagus and saute for 4-5 minutes, stirring occasionally, until tender. Remove from heat and set side.
2. Meanwhile, in a large mixing bowl, combine the kale and lemony dressing. Then use your fingers to massage the dressing into the kale for 2-3 minutes, or until the leaves are dark and softened. Add the Brussels sprouts, quinoa, and cooked asparagus, and toss until combined.
3. To assemble the bowls, smear a spoonful of hummus along the side of each bowl. Then portion the kale salad evenly between the four bowls, top with avocado, egg, and your desired garnishes. Serve immediately.

To Make The Lemon Vinaigrette:

1. Whisk all ingredients together in a small mixing bowl until combined.

4. Amazing Mexican Casserole

Prep Time: 20 Minutes

Cook Time: 55 Minutes

Servings: 12

Ingredients

- Pounds ground sausage or Mexican chorizo
- 1 small white onion, peeled and diced
- 1 poblano or green bell pepper, cored and diced
- 4 cloves garlic, minced
- 1 (15-ounce) jar red or green salsa (approx. 2 cups)
- 1 (15-ounce) can black or pinto beans, rinsed and drained
- 2/3 cup whole-kernel corn, frozen or canned
- 1 teaspoon ground cumin
- 1 teaspoon fine sea salt
- 12 large eggs
- 1/3 cup milk
- 8 corn tortillas, halved
- 3 cups shredded Mexican-blend cheese

- Optional toppings: diced avocado, diced red onion, chopped fresh cilantro, diced green onion, sliced fresh jalapeños, and/or crumbled cotija cheese

Instructions

2. Heat oven to 400°F. Lightly mist a 9 x 13-inch baking dish with cooking spray; set aside.
3. Cook the sausage in a large sauté pan over medium-high heat until browned, crumbling the sausage as it cooks. Use a slotted spoon to transfer the sausage to a clean plate, reserving a tablespoon or so of grease in the sauté pan. (Or if there is no grease remaining, add a tablespoon of oil to the pan.)
4. Add the onion and pepper and sauté for 5 minutes, stirring occasionally, until softened. Add the garlic and sauté for 1-2 minutes more, stirring occasionally, until fragrant.
5. Add in the salsa, beans, corn, cumin, salt, cooked sausage, and stir until the mixture is completely combined. Remove pan from the heat, and set aside.
6. In a separate bowl, whisk together the eggs and milk until evenly combined; set aside.

7. Alright, time to layer up all of the ingredients! Layer half of the tortillas in an even layer in the bottom of the baking dish. Then top evenly with half of the sausage mixture, half of the egg mixture, and half of the cheese. Repeat with another layer of tortillas, sausage mixture, egg mixture and cheese.

8. Cover the dish with foil and bake for 45-50 minutes*, or until the center of the casserole is cooked through and no longer jiggly (or when a toothpick inserted in the center of the casserole comes out clean).

9. Transfer baking dish to a wire cooling rack and let cool for 10 minutes. Then sprinkle with your desired toppings, slice and serve warm!

5. Cozy Autumn Casserole

Prep Time: 20 Minutes

Cook Time: 50 Minutes

Servings: 12

Ingredients

- 8 ounces baby bella mushrooms, quartered
- 1.5 pounds potatoes, diced into 1/2-inch cubes (I used half sweet potatoes, half Yukon gold)
- 1 large red bell pepper, cored and diced
- 1 medium white or yellow onion, peeled and diced
- 3 tablespoons olive oil
- Sea salt and freshly-cracked black pepper
- 1 pound ground Italian sausage (or breakfast sausage)
- 4 cloves garlic, peeled and minced
- 2 handfuls roughly-chopped fresh kale, tough stems discarded
- 15 eggs, whisked
- 2/3 cup milk
- 1 1/2 tablespoons Old Bay Seasoning, or more/less to taste

Instructions

1. Prep oven and baking pan. Heat oven to 400°F. Line a large baking sheet (or two medium baking sheets) with parchment paper; set aside. Lightly mist a 9 x 13-inch baking pan with cooking spray; set aside.

2. Roast the vegetables. Spread the mushrooms, potatoes, red bell pepper, and onion out on a large baking sheet (or two medium baking sheets). Drizzle evenly with the oil, and season with a few generous pinches of salt and pepper. Toss the veggies until they are evenly coated with the oil and arranged in an even layer, not overlapping. Bake for about 20-25 minutes, or until the potatoes are tender. Remove baking sheet(s) from the oven, and carefully transfer the veggies into the prepared baking dish; set aside.

3. Brown the sausage. Meanwhile, as the veggies are roasting, cook the sausage in a large sauté pan over medium-high heat until browned, using a wooden spoon to break up and crumble the sausage as it cooks. Once the sausage is browned, add in the garlic and kale and sauté for an extra 2-3 minutes, stirring occasionally, until fragrant. (If there is not leftover oil in the pan from the sausage, you may need to add in an extra teaspoon or two to sauté the garlic and kale.)

Remove pan from heat, and transfer the sausage into the prepared baking dish; set aside.

4. Whisk the eggs. In a separate large bowl or measuring cup, whisk together the eggs, milk, Old Bay seasoning, plus an extra 1 teaspoon salt and 1/2 teaspoon black pepper until combined.

5. Assemble the casserole. Once the veggies and sausage have been cooked and added to the baking dish, use a spoon to give them a brief toss. Then spread the mixture out in an even layer in the baking dish. Carefully pour the whisked egg mixture evenly on top of the veggies and sausage.

6. Bake. Bake uncovered for 30-35 minutes, or until a toothpick inserted in the middle of the casserole comes out completely clean. (If the veggies on top of the casserole get too browned before the casserole is done, just lay a piece of aluminum foil gently on top of the baking dish until the inside is cooked through.) Remove from the oven and transfer to a cooling rack to cool for 10 minutes.

7. Serve warm. Then slice, serve, and enjoy! Or cover and refrigerate for up to 3 days.

6. Easy Tacos

Prep Time: 15 Minutes

Cook Time: 15 Minutes

Servings: 8

Ingredients

- 8 small corn or flour tortillas
- 8 large eggs, either scrambled or fried
- 1 batch homemade refried beans
- 2 avocados, peeled, pitted and sliced
- Your choice of salsa: red, green, or pico de gallo
- Your choice of toppings: chopped fresh cilantro, cheese, sour cream and/or diced jalapeños

Instructions

1. Prepare the refried beans in a large saucepan according to recipe instructions.
2. Meanwhile, as the beans are cooking, go ahead and scramble (see below) or fry the eggs in a non-stick sauté pan.

3. Once the beans and eggs are ready to go, it's time to assemble the tacos! Simply spread a spoonful of refried beans on a tortilla, top with a spoonful of scrambled eggs, then load it up with avocado, salsa and any of your preferred toppings.

4. Serve immediately and enjoy!

7. Black Bean Tacos

Prep Time: 10 Minutes

Cook Time: 10 Minutes

Servings: 10

Ingredients

Black Bean Tacos Ingredients:

- 1 batch zesty Mexican black beans
- 1 batch scrambled eggs
- 8–10 small wheat or corn tortillas
- Toppings: chopped fresh cilantro, diced red onions, diced avocado, crumbled queso fresco (or shredded Pepper Jack cheese), fresh lime wedges, and/or salsa

Zesty Black Beans Ingredients:

- 1 tablespoon avocado oil (or olive oil, or any other mild-flavored oil)
- 1 cup diced white or red onions
- 1 jalapeño, finely-diced (with seeds removed)
- 5 cloves garlic, peeled and minced
- 2 (15-ounce) cans black beans, rinsed and drained
- 1 1/2 teaspoons ground cumin

- Juice of 1 small lime
- Salt and pepper

Scrambled Eggs Ingredients:

- 10 eggs
- 1/3 cup milk
- Salt and pepper

Instructions

To Make The Black Bean Breakfast Tacos:

1. Prepare the zesty black beans and scrambled eggs. (And I recommend prepping your toppings while those cook, to save time.)
2. Once all of your fillings and toppings are ready to go, fill your tortillas with a large spoonful (each) of the black bean mixture and scrambled eggs. Then sprinkle on your desired toppings. Serve immediately.

To Make The Zesty Black Beans:

1. Heat oil in a medium saucepan over medium-high heat. Add the onion and jalapeno, and saute for 4-5 minutes, stirring occasionally, until the onion is cooked and soft and translucent. Stir in the garlic and saute

for 1-2 minutes, stirring occasionally, until fragrant. Stir in the black beans, cumin and lime until completely combined. Saute for 1-2 minutes, or until the black beans are warmed through.

2. Season to taste with salt and pepper, then remove from the heat and serve.

To Make The Scrambled Eggs:

1. Whisk together eggs and milk and a pinch of salt and pepper in a large bowl until smooth.

2. Heat a large saute pan over medium-heat, and spray with cooking spray (or melt a tablespoon of butter in the bottom of the pan). Add the egg mixture and cook, stirring frequently, until the eggs are scrambled and cooked through. Remove from heat and serve.

8. Reuben Sandwich on Pumpernickel English Muffins

Prep Time: 2hrs 5 Minutes

Cook Time: 30 Minutes

Servings: 12

Ingredients

Reuben Breakfast Sandwich:

- 2 Whole Eggs
- 1 Tbsp Butter
- 4 large slices Pastrami
- ½ cup Sauerkraut
- ¼ cup Mayo
- 2 Tbsp Ketchup
- ¼ tsp Horseradish puree
- 2 Pumpernickel English Muffins

English Muffins:

- 2 Tablespoons Vegetable Oil, For Greasing Bowl
- 4 ounces, fluid Water, between 100-105 Degrees
- 7 ounces, fluid Milk, between 100-105 Degrees
- ? Ounces, weight Instant Dry Yeast
- 2 Tablespoons Butter, Divided

- 1/2 pound Flour, All Purpose
- ½ pound Rye Flour
- 2 Tbsp Molasses
- 1 Tsp Cocoa Powder
- ½ tsp Caraway Seeds
- 1 teaspoon Salt
- ½ cups Cornmeal for Working Dough

Instructions

To Make The Reuben Sandwiches:

1. Mix together mayo, ketchup and horseradish. Slice english muffins and toast.
2. In large skillet, sauté pastrami until heated through and browned slightly. Heat sauerkraut until hot. Remove pastrami and kraut and set aside.
3. Add butter to the pan and fry two eggs until just set. Slater mayo/ketchup/horseradish mixture onto english muffins, top with pastrami, kraut and fried egg. Promptly devour.

To Make The English Muffins:

1. Grease a large mixing bowl with vegetable oil. Set aside. Line a large rimmed baking sheet with parchment paper or a silicone liner. Set aside.

2. In the bowl of a stand mixer, whisk together water, milk, yeast, 1 tablespoon of butter (melted and cooled to between 100-105°F) and 5 ounces of flour. Cover with plastic wrap and let sit for 30 minutes to form a "sponge" or "starter" for muffins.

3. Once the sponge has doubled in size, attach dough hook to the stand mixer along with the bowl. Turn on low and add in remaining flours, cocoa powder and molasses to the sponge that was formed. Add in salt and caraway seeds. Allow to mix on medium and knead until satin and smooth, approximately 5 minutes. When kneading is complete, scrape dough from mixer bowl and transfer to greased bowl that had been set aside. Cover with plastic wrap and allow to rise 45 minutes to 1 hour.

4. Preheat your oven to 375°F. Dust a clean and sanitized countertop or work surface with cornmeal. Turn out dough from greased bowl and stretch evenly until it is about 3/4? Thick. Handle dough lightly so it does not become tough.

5. With a 4? Round biscuit cutter, cut out as many rounds as possible. Place them on parchment or silicone lined baking sheet. Re-roll dough to obtain more muffin rounds. But do not re-roll more than once.

6. In a large skillet, heat remaining 1 tablespoon of butter to coat the pan on about medium heat. Lightly brown each side of each muffin, about 1 minute per side. Place each muffin back onto lined baking sheet until all have been browned.

7. Place in heated oven for 15-20 minute until cooked through. Immediately cool on a wire rack when completely cooked. Serve warm with jam of your choice and devour.

8. The muffins can be frozen to preserve or eaten within 4 days.

9. Crunchy Granola

Prep Time: 10 Minutes

Cook Time: 40 Minutes

Servings: 10

Ingredients

- 5 cups rolled oats
- 1/2 cup ground flax seed (optional)
- 2 to 3 cups raw almonds or pecan halves, or a mixture
- ¾ cup light brown sugar
- 1 Tbsp. ground cinnamon
- 1 tsp. ground ginger
- 1 tsp. salt
- 1 cup unsweetened apple sauce
- 1/2 cup honey
- 2 tsp. vanilla
- 2 tbsp. vegetable oil
- 1 cup. Favorite dried fruit (cherries, cranberries, raisins, apricots, etc.)

Instructions

1. Set racks in the upper and lower thirds of the oven.
   Preheat the oven to 300°F.

2. In a large bowl, combine all of the dry ingredients. Stir
   to mix well. In a small bowl, combine all of the wet
   ingredients. Stir to mix well. Pour the wet ingredients
   over the dry ones, and stir well.

3. Spread the mixture evenly on two rimmed baking
   sheets, either greased with cooking spray or covered
   with parchment paper. Bake for 35 to 40 minutes, or
   until evenly golden brown. Set a timer to go off every
   ten minutes while the granola bakes, so you can rotate
   the pans and give the granola a good stir; this helps it
   to cook evenly.

4. When its ready, remove the pans from the oven, stir
   well – this will keep it from cooling into a hard, solid
   sheet – and set aside to cool. The finished granola may
   still feel slightly soft when it comes out of the oven, but
   it will crisp as it cools.

5. Scoop cooled granola into to a large zipper-lock plastic
   bag or other airtight container. Store in the refrigerator
   indefinitely.

10. No Bake Energy Bites

Prep Time: 20 Minutes

Cook Time: 00 Minutes

Servings: 23

Ingredients

- 1 cup old-fashioned oats
- 2/3 cup toasted shredded coconut (sweetened or unsweetened)
- 1/2 cup creamy peanut butter
- 1/2 cup ground flaxseed
- 1/2 cup semisweet chocolate chips (or vegan chocolate chips)
- 1/3 cup honey
- 1 tablespoon chia seeds (optional)
- 1 teaspoon vanilla extract

Instructions

1. Stir everything together. Stir all ingredients together in a large mixing bowl until thoroughly combined.

2. Chill. Cover the mixing bowl and chill in the refrigerator for 1-2 hours, or until the mixture is chilled. (This will help the mixture stick together more easily.)

3. Roll into balls. Roll into mixture into 1-inch balls.

4. Serve. Then enjoy immediately! Or refrigerate in a sealed container for up to 1 week, or freeze for up to 3 months.

LUNCH

11. Poblano White Chicken Chili

Prep Time: 10 Minutes

Cook Time: 20 Minutes

Servings: 3

Ingredients

- 1 tablespoon olive oil

- 1 small white onion, peeled and diced

- 2 large poblano peppers, cored and diced

- 4 cloves garlic, minced

- 8 cups chicken stock

- 1 tablespoon ground cumin

- 1 teaspoon chili powder

- 3 (15-ounce) cans white or pinto beans, rinsed and drained

- 3 cups (about 1 pound) diced or shredded cooked chicken

- Fine sea salt and freshly-cracked black pepper

- Toppings: chopped fresh cilantro, diced avocado, diced red or green onions, fresh lime wedges, grated or crumbled cheese, sliced jalapeños, sour cream, tortilla strips

Instructions

1. Sauté the veggies. Heat oil in a large stockpot over medium-high heat. Add the onion and poblano peppers and sauté for 5 minutes, stirring occasionally, until softened. Add the garlic and sauté for 1-2 more minutes, stirring frequently, until fragrant.
2. Add the next round of ingredients. Add the chicken stock, ground cumin, chili powder and stir to combine.
3. Blend the beans. While the soup is heating, ladle out about 1 cup of the soup and transfer it to a blender. Add one (rinsed and drained) can of beans to the blender too, then purée until smooth.
4. Add the remaining ingredients. Add the purée, chicken, and the remaining 2 cans of beans to the soup and stir to combine. Continue cooking until the soup reaches a simmer. Then reduce heat to medium-low to maintain the simmer and cook for 5 more minutes.
5. Season. Taste the soup and season with salt and pepper as needed.

6. Serve. Serve warm, garnished with lots (and lots!) of
    your favorite toppings.

12. Homemade Buttermilk Biscuits

Prep Time: 30 Minutes

Cook Time: 10 Minutes

Servings: 8

Ingredients

- 2 cups (284 grams) all-purpose flour
- 1 tablespoon baking powder
- 1 tablespoon light brown sugar
- 1 teaspoon fine sea salt
- 1/4 teaspoon baking soda
- 6 tablespoons (85 grams) very cold butter, diced into 1/2-inch cubes
- 1 cup cold buttermilk
- Optional toppings: extra melted butter and flaky sea salt

Instructions

1. Mix the dry ingredients: Combine the flour, baking powder, brown sugar, salt and baking soda in a large mixing bowl. Stir briefly to combine.

2. Cut in the butter. Sprinkle the diced butter over the dry ingredient mixture. Use a pastry cutter or two forks (or a food processor*) to cut the butter into the dry ingredients until it is well-mixed and forms pea-sized chunks of butter.

3. Add the buttermilk. Pour in the cold buttermilk and stir until the dough until it is just combined. (Try to avoid over-mixing the dough.)

4. Form the dough. Turn the dough out onto a floured work surface. Use your hands to quickly shape the dough into a small rectangle. Use a rolling pin to roll the dough out evenly until it is about 1/2-inch thick.

5. Fold the dough. Then fold the dough on top of itself into thirds (like you are folding an envelope, see image above). Rotate the dough 90 degrees. Then repeat the folding process a second time, rotate, repeat the folding process a third time, rotate.

6. Cut the dough. Roll the dough out once more into a roughly 10 x 5-inch rectangle. Then use a 2 to 2.5-inch biscuit cutter to firmly cut the dough into 8 circles, taking care not to twist the biscuit cutter at all when cutting the dough, and arrange the biscuits evenly on the prepared baking sheet. If you would like, re-roll the

remaining dough scraps and cut out 1 or 2 more biscuits.

7. Heat the oven. Heat the oven to 450°F (232°C). And transfer the biscuits to your freezer or refrigerator for 15 minutes as the oven heats.

8. Bake. Once the oven is ready to go, bake the biscuits for 10-12 minutes, or until they achieve your desired level of browning on top. Transfer the baking sheet to a wire rack. Then, if you would like, brush the tops of the biscuits with some melted butter and sprinkle with a pinch of flaky sea salt.

9. Serve. Serve warm and enjoy!

13. Peanut Curry Lentil Soup

Prep Time: 30 Minutes

Cook Time: 10 Minutes

Servings: 8

Ingredients

- 1 tablespoon olive oil
- 1 medium yellow onion, diced
- 1 yellow bell pepper, diced
- 4 cloves garlic, minced
- 5 to 6 cups vegetable broth
- 1 1/4 pounds sweet potatoes, peeled and diced into ¾-inch cubes
- 3/4 cup brown lentils
- 2 tablespoons Thai red curry paste
- 1 (15-ounce) can full-fat coconut milk
- 2 cups chopped fresh kale
- 2 tablespoons natural creamy peanut butter
- 2 tablespoons lime juice (approximately 1 lime)
- Fine sea salt and freshly-ground black pepper
- Toppings: chopped fresh cilantro and finely-chopped peanuts

Instructions

1. Sauté the veggies. Heat oil in a large stockpot over medium-high heat. Add the onion and bell pepper and sauté for 5 minutes, stirring occasionally. Add the garlic and sauté for 1-2 minutes, stirring frequently, until fragrant.

2. Simmer. Add the vegetable broth, sweet potatoes, and lentils, curry paste and stir to combine. Continue cooking until the soup reaches a simmer. Then reduce heat to medium-low (or whatever temperature is needed to maintain a low simmer), cover, and cook for about 20 to 25 minutes or until both the lentils and sweet potatoes are tender.

3. Finish. Stir in the coconut milk, kale, peanut butter and lime juice until completely combined. Taste and season the soup with salt and pepper, if needed. Feel free to also add in more curry paste or peanut butter to taste.

4. Serve. Serve warm, garnished with cilantro and chopped peanuts, and enjoy!

14. Mango Lentil Salad

Prep Time: 5 Minutes

Cook Time: 25 Minutes

Servings: 4

Ingredients

- 1 cup dried lentils, rinsed and picked over
- 1 large avocado, diced
- 1 large mango, diced
- Half a medium red onion, finely diced
- 1 cup chopped fresh baby spinach
- 1 cup chopped fresh mint
- 2/3 cup chopped almonds
- 2/3 cup crumbled feta cheese
- 1 batch everyday salad dressing
- Fine sea salt and freshly-ground black pepper

Instructions

1. Cook the lentils. Cook the lentils in lightly-salted water according to package directions until tender. Pour into

a fine-mesh strainer and rinse with cold water until chilled, then drain off any extra water.

2. Toss. Combine the lentils, avocado, mango, red onion, baby spinach, mint, almonds and feta in a large mixing bowl and drizzle evenly with the dressing. Toss gently until combined. Taste and season with salt and pepper as needed.

3. Serve. Serve immediately and enjoy!

15. Tuna Avocado Brown Rice Bowls

Prep Time: 5 Minutes

Cook Time: 30 Minutes

Servings: 4

Ingredients

Tuna Avocado Rice Bowl Ingredients

- 1 1/2 cups uncooked brown rice

- 3 ounces feta cheese, crumbled

- 2 (5-ounce) cans tuna packed in oil, drained

- 2 medium avocados, diced

- Half of an English cucumber, diced

- Half of a small red onion, very thinly sliced

- 1/4 cup chopped fresh dill, loosely packed

Sumac Dressing Ingredients

- 2 tablespoons olive oil

- 2 tablespoons lemon juice

- 1 teaspoon Dijon mustard

- 1/2 teaspoon each: fine sea salt, freshly-ground black pepper, ground cumin, ground sumac

Instructions

1. Cook the brown rice. Cook the brown rice however you prefer, either on the stovetop, in the Instant Pot or in a rice cooker (per appliance instructions).
2. Make the dressing. Whisk all ingredients together in a bowl (or shake together in a sealed jar) until emulsified.
3. Make the tuna salad. Add the feta, drained tuna, avocado, cucumber, red onion and dill to a large mixing bowl. Drizzle evenly with the dressing, then toss gently until evenly combined.
4. Serve. Serve immediately over brown rice, garnished with extra feta, dill, ground sumac and black pepper if desired.

16. Garlic Chili Oil Noodles with Shrimp

Prep Time: 10 Minutes

Cook Time: 15 Minutes

Servings: 4

Ingredients

Shrimp Noodle Stir-Fry Ingredients:

- 1 pound jumbo raw shrimp, peeled and deveined
- Fine sea salt and freshly-ground black pepper
- 1/3 cup avocado oil (or any neutral oil), divided
- 4 baby bok choy, halved vertically
- 8 ounces uncooked wide knife-cut noodles (or your choice of noodles)
- 6 large garlic cloves, minced
- 2 scallions, thinly sliced (white and green parts separated)
- 1 tablespoon minced fresh ginger

Chili Oil Mix Ingredients:

- 2 tablespoons low-sodium soy sauce
- 2 tablespoons sesame seeds
- 1 to 2 tablespoons gochugaru flakes (or powder)

- 1 tablespoon Chinese black vinegar

- 1 teaspoon granulated white sugar

- 1/4 teaspoon fine sea salt

Instructions

1. Prep the water. Bring a large pot of water to a boil.

2. Prep the chili oil mix. Meanwhile, in a small mixing bowl, whisk together all of the chili oil mix ingredients until combined.

3. Cook the shrimp. Season the shrimp generously with salt and pepper. Heat 1 tablespoon oil to a large non-stick sauté pan over medium-high heat. Add the shrimp in an even layer (you may need to do this in two batches, depending on the size of your pan) and sauté for 1-2 minutes per side until the shrimp are no longer pink and cooked through. Transfer the cooked shrimp to a clean plate and set aside.

4. Cook the bok choy. Add 1 more tablespoon oil to the pan. Place the bok choy halves cut-side-down in the pan. Cook for 1 minute or until lightly golden on the bottom, then flip and cook for 30 seconds on the other side. Transfer the cooked bok choy to a clean plate and set aside.

5. Cook the noodles. Add the noodles to the boiling water and cook according to package instructions until al dente.

6. Cook the garlic chili oil. While the noodles are cooking, add the remaining 1/4 cup oil to the pan. Add the garlic, ginger and the white parts of the scallions and sauté for 1-2 minutes, or until the garlic begins to turn lightly golden. Immediately pour the chili oil mix into the pan (be careful, as it will bubble up intensely) and stir to combine. Remove pan from heat until the noodles are ready.

7. Combine. Strain the noodles and add them immediately to the pan with the sauce. Add the cooked shrimp and green parts of the scallions and toss everything together until evenly combined.

8. Serve. Serve immediately with the cooked bok choy and enjoy!

17. Spicy Sesame Gochujang Noodles

Prep Time: 15 Minutes

Cook Time: 15 Minutes

Servings: 6

Ingredients

Noodle Stir-Fry Ingredients:

- 8 ounces thin rice noodles
- 2 tablespoons olive oil, divided
- 1 pound boneless skinless chicken breasts, thinly sliced into bite-sized pieces
- Fine sea salt and freshly-ground black pepper
- 8 ounces shiitake mushrooms, thinly sliced
- 4 scallions, sliced into 1.5-inch pieces
- 2 cloves garlic, minced
- 2 handfuls baby spinach
- Optional toppings: chopped fresh cilantro or Thai basil, chopped peanuts, toasted sesame seeds, lime wedges

Sesame Gochujang Sauce Ingredients:

- 1/2 cup water

- 1/4 cup gochujang paste

- 2 tablespoons low-sodium soy sauce

- 1 1/2 tablespoons maple syrup or honey

- 2 teaspoons toasted sesame oil

- Juice of one lime (about 2 tablespoons)

Instructions

1. Prep the rice noodles. Soak the rice noodles according to package instructions until they are just under al dente (you still want them to have a bit of bite), then drain and set aside.

2. Mix the gochujang sauce. Meanwhile, as the noodles are soaking, whisk all of the sauce ingredients together in a measuring cup until evenly combined.

3. Cook the chicken. Season the chicken with salt and pepper. Heat 1 tablespoon oil in a large sauté pan or wok over medium-high heat. Add the sliced chicken and sauté for 4 to 5 minutes, stirring occasionally, until browned and cooked through. Transfer the chicken to a clean plate and set aside.

4. Cook the veggies. Add the remaining 1 tablespoon oil to the hot pan along with the mushrooms and white parts of the scallions. Sauté for 5 to 7 minutes, stirring

occasionally, until the mushrooms are browned. Add in the garlic sauté for 2 more minutes, stirring frequently.

5. Combine. Add the cooked noodles, chicken, sauce, spinach and the green parts of the scallions to the sauté pan. Gently toss the mixture until it is evenly combined and the spinach has wilted and the noodles are heated through. If the mixture seems dry at any point, add in some extra water (up to 1 cup) to help thin out the sauce. Taste and season with extra soy sauce, if needed.

6. Serve. Serve warm, garnished with an extra lime wedge and any other toppings that sound good. Enjoy!

18. Greek Salmon Salad Bowls

Prep Time: 15 Minutes

Cook Time: 10 Minutes

Servings: 2

Ingredients

- 1 pound salmon filets
- Fine sea salt and freshly-cracked black pepper
- 1 tablespoon olive oil
- 2 ounces fresh arugula
- 1 large red bell pepper, chopped into bite-sized pieces
- Half of an English cucumber, sliced into bite-sized pieces
- Half of a small red onion, thinly sliced
- 2/3 cup roasted pepitas
- 1/2 cup crumbled feta cheese
- 1 batch Everyday Dressing
- 1 avocado, sliced or diced

Instructions

1. Cook the salmon. Season the salmon with a few generous pinches of salt and pepper. Heat the olive oil in a large non-stick sauté pan. Place the salmon filets flesh-side down and cook undisturbed for about 3-4 minutes, or until golden. Flip and cook the other side for about 2-4 more minutes, until the salmon reaches your desired level of doneness and flakes easily with a fork. (Cooking time will also depend on the thickness of the salmon.) Transfer salmon to a clean plate and set aside.

2. Toss. Combine the arugula, bell pepper, cucumber, red onion, pepitas, feta and cooked salmon in a large mixing bowl. Drizzle evenly with the dressing, then gently toss to combine.

3. Serve. Serve immediately, topped with the avocado plus extra feta and/or pepitas, for garnish.

19. Rainbow Peanut Noodles

Prep Time: 25 Minutes

Cook Time: 10 Minutes

Servings: 6

Ingredients

Rainbow Pasta Ingredients:

- 12 ounces whole wheat pasta (or soba, ramen, or rice noodles)
- 3 scallions, thinly sliced
- 2 small bell peppers, cored and very thinly sliced (I used one red, one yellow)
- 1 cup julienned carrots
- 1 cup shredded red cabbage
- 1 cup chopped fresh cilantro (loosely packed)
- Optional toppings: finely chopped peanuts, cilantro, green onions, lime wedges, and/or toasted sesame seeds

Peanut Sauce Ingredients:

- 1/2 cup natural creamy peanut butter
- 1/4 cup low-sodium soy sauce

- 1/4 cup lime juice

- 2 tablespoons toasted sesame oil

- 1 to 2 tablespoons honey, to taste

- 1 tablespoon chili garlic sauce

- 1 tablespoon grated fresh ginger

- 1 large clove garlic, pressed or finely minced

Instructions

1. Make the peanut sauce. Whisk together all ingredients in a small mixing bowl until combined. Taste and sweeten with additional honey if desired.

2. Cook the pasta. Cook the pasta in a large stockpot of salted boiling water until just barely al dente. (Try to avoid overcooking the noodles.) Transfer 1/2 cup of the starchy hot water to the peanut sauce. Reserve an additional 1/2 cup of the starchy water and set it aside for later. Drain the pasta, then return it to the large stockpot.

3. Toss. Add the scallions, bell peppers, carrots, cabbage, cilantro, peanuts and peanut sauce to the pot. Toss gently until everything is coated evenly in the sauce. If the sauce seems too dry, add in some of the reserved starchy water and toss to combine.

4. Serve. Serve warm, garnished with your favorite toppings.

20. French Lentil and Mushroom Soup

Prep Time: 15 Minutes

Cook Time: 45 Minutes

Servings: 8

Ingredients

- 1 tablespoon olive oil
- 2 large leeks (white and light green parts only), halved and sliced
- 2 celery stalks, diced
- 1 pound baby bella mushrooms, sliced
- 5 large cloves garlic
- 2/3 cup dry white wine
- 8 cups vegetable stock
- 4 sprigs fresh thyme
- 2 bay leaves
- 2 cups French lentils, rinsed and drained
- 3 large handfuls of baby spinach (or chopped kale or collard greens)
- 2 tablespoons balsamic vinegar
- Fine sea salt and freshly-cracked black pepper

Instructions

1. Sauté the veggies. Heat the olive oil in a large stockpot over medium-high heat. Add the leeks, celery, mushrooms, and sauté for 6-8 minutes, stirring occasionally. Add the garlic and sauté for 2 minutes, stirring occasionally. Pour in the white wine and deglaze the pan by using a wooden spoon to gently lift up any brown bits that have stuck to the bottom of the pan.

2. Simmer. Add in the vegetable stock, thyme and bay leaves and stir to combine. Continue cooking until the soup reaches a simmer. Add in the lentils and stir to combine. Then reduce heat to medium-low, cover, and simmer for 30 minutes or until the lentils are tender, checking back occasionally to stir the soup so that the lentils do not stick to the bottom of the pot.

3. Season. Remove and discard the thyme sprigs and bay leaves. Stir in the spinach and balsamic until the spinach begins to wilt. Then give the soup a taste and season with however much salt, black pepper, and/or extra balsamic you think is needed.

4. Serve. Serve the soup warm, garnished with an extra crack of black pepper (I also sprinkled some microgreens on top of mine), and enjoy!

DINNER

21. Spicy Black Bean Soup

Prep Time: 5 Minutes

Cook Time: 20 Minutes

Servings: 5

Ingredients

- 2 Tbsp. olive oil
- 1 medium yellow onion, chopped
- 1 red or orange bell pepper, cored and chopped
- 1 carrot, chopped
- 3 cloves garlic, minced
- Half a jalapeno, seeded and diced
- 2 cups chicken broth (or vegetable broth)
- 2 (15 oz.) cans black beans
- 1 (14.5 oz) can diced tomatoes with green chiles (Rotel)
- 1 bay leaf
- 1 tsp. cumin
- 1 tsp. chipotle powder
- 1 tsp. kosher salt
- 1/4 tsp. cayenne

- Optional garnish: sour cream, chopped fresh cilantro, chopped bell peppers, shredded cheese, crumbled tortilla chips, diced avocados

Instructions

1. Heat olive oil in a large stockpot over medium-high heat. Add onion and cook for 3 minutes. Add bell pepper, carrot, garlic and jalapeno, and continue cooking another 5 minutes or until the onion is translucent. Add remaining eight ingredients (chicken broth through cayenne), and stir to combine. Bring to a boil, then reduce heat to medium-low and let soup simmer for at least 10 minutes.

2. You can either serve this soup as is, or use an immersion blender or a traditional blender (blending in small batches) to puree the soup. Serve warm, and garnish with suggested ingredients if desired.

22. One Hour Rosemary Garlic Rolls

Prep Time: 45 Minutes

Cook Time: 15 Minutes

Servings: 12

Ingredients

Dinner Rolls Ingredients:

- 1 cup water
- 2 tablespoons melted butter
- 1/2 cup milk
- 2 tablespoons honey
- 1 tablespoon active-dry yeast
- 3 1/2 to 4 cups all-purpose flour
- 1 tablespoon finely chopped fresh rosemary
- 1 teaspoon fine sea salt
- 1 teaspoon garlic powder
- Optional: flaky sea salt, for serving

Garlic Herb Butter Ingredients:

- 3 tablespoons butter
- 2 cloves garlic, peeled and thinly sliced
- 1 tablespoon finely chopped fresh parsley

Instructions

1. Heat the liquids. Stir together the water and melted butter in a saucepan, then add in the milk and honey and stir until combined. Heat the mixture over medium low heat, stirring occasionally, until it reaches 110°F. It will be warm but not hot to the touch. (Alternately, you can heat the mixture in a microwave until it reaches 110°F.)

2. Add yeast. Pour the liquid mixture into the large bowl of a stand mixer (or see instructions below for how to knead by hand). Sprinkle the yeast on top and give it a quick stir combine, then let the yeast activate for 5 minutes until it is foamy.

3. Mix in dry ingredients. Add in 3 1/2 cups of flour (not all of the flour), rosemary, and fine sea salt and garlic powder. Using the dough-hook, beat the dough on medium-low speed until combined. If the dough is sticking to the sides of the bowl, add in 1/4 cup more flour at a time (no more than 4 cups total) until the dough pulls away from the sides of the bowl and is only slightly sticky to the touch. Continue mixing on low speed for 4-5 minutes until the dough is smooth.

4. Let the dough rise. Form the dough into a ball with your hands and transfer it to a greased bowl. Cover the

bowl with a damp towel or foil, and let it rise briefly in a warm location for 15 minutes.

5. Prep your oven and baking dish. Heat the oven to 400°F. Grease a 9 x 13-inch baking dish and set aside.

6. Form the rolls. Gently punch the dough down and divide it into 15 equal-sized pieces. Form each piece into a ball and place the dough balls in the greased baking dish. Cover the dish with a damp towel or foil and let the dough balls rise for an additional 15-20 minutes.

7. Bake. Uncover and bake for 15 to 20 minutes or until the tops of the rolls are browned to your liking, then transfer the pan to a wire baking rack.

8. Make the garlic butter. While the rolls are baking, melt the butter in a small saucepan over low heat. Add the sliced garlic and simmer for 2 minutes, then remove the pan from heat, strain out and discard the garlic slices. Stir in the chopped parsley until combined.

9. Serve warm. Brush the hot rolls with the garlic butter and sprinkle with a pinch of flaky sea salt. Serve warm and enjoy!

23. Cranberry-Pomegranate Sauce

Prep Time: 2 Minutes

Cook Time: 20 Minutes

Servings: 4

Ingredients

- 1 bag (12 oz.) fresh cranberries
- 2 cups (16 oz.) POM pomegranate juice
- 1/2 – 3/4 cups sugar (depending on your preferred level of sweetness)
- Seeds from 1 pomegranate (optional)

Instructions

1. Combine the cranberries, pomegranate juice and sugar together in a medium saucepan over medium-high heat. Bring to a boil, and then reduce heat to medium-low and simmer for 20 minutes, stirring occasionally to prevent burning.

2. Then remove from heat, and stir in pomegranate seeds. Refrigerate until ready to serve (and sauce will thicken as it cools).

24. Five Spice Tofu with Sesame Noodles

Prep Time: 35 Minutes

Cook Time: 10 Minutes

Servings: 8

Ingredients

Five Spice Tofu Ingredients:

- 1 pound block of extra-firm tofu
- 2 tablespoons olive oil
- 1/2 cup hoisin sauce
- 2 tablespoons rice vinegar
- 1 tablespoon five spice powder
- Toppings: toasted sesame seeds and thinly-sliced green onions

Sesame Noodles Ingredients:

- 1 pound uncooked pasta noodles
- 1/4 cup low-sodium soy sauce
- 2 tablespoons rice vinegar
- 1 tablespoon toasted sesame oil
- 1 teaspoon ground ginger
- 1/2 teaspoon chili garlic sauce or sriracha

- 1/2 teaspoon garlic powder
- 1/4 teaspoon freshly-cracked black pepper
- 1/2 cup thinly-sliced green onions

Instructions

1. Press the tofu. Slice the block of tofu into 1/2-inch slabs. Lay some paper towels or a clean tea towel on a flat surface, and place the slabs side by side on top of the paper towels. Cover with another layer of paper towels, then place a cutting board on top of the tofu, and stack a bunch of heavy cans or pots or whatever you can safely balance on the cutting board. Let the tofu drain for at least 15-30 minutes.
2. Make the five spice sauce. Whisk together the hoisin, rice vinegar and five spice powder until combined. Set aside.
3. Make the sesame noodles. Make the sesame noodles according to recipe instructions here.
4. Cook the tofu. Remove the paper towels and slice the tofu into 1/2-inch cubes. Heat the oil in a large non-stick sauté pan over medium-high heat. Add the tofu and sauté for 8-10 minutes, flipping and tossing the tofu every 2 or so minutes, until it is crispy and

browned. Remove pan from heat, add hoisin sauce, and toss until combined.

5. Serve. Serve the sesame noodles topped with the tofu (plus any extra veggies you might like to add), sprinkled with toasted sesame seeds and thinly-sliced green onions for garnish. Enjoy!!

25. Roasted Vegetable & Black Bean Tacos

Prep Time: 5 Minutes

Cook Time: 25 Minutes

Servings: 5

Ingredients

- Diced vegetables (I used red/yellow bell peppers, sweet potatoes, poblanos, onions, and mushrooms)
- Canola or vegetable oil
- Salt and freshly-cracked black pepper
- Corn tortillas
- Black beans, drained (if from a can)
- Optional toppings: chopped cilantro, sour cream, shredded cheese, guacamole, etc.

Instructions

1. Preheat oven to 425 degrees. Line a baking sheet with aluminum foil.
2. Toss the vegetables in oil (about 1 Tbsp. oil for every 4 cups of veggies). Then spread out in a single layer on the prepared baking sheet, and season with salt and

freshly-ground black pepper. Roast for about 20-25 minutes, until veggies are soft and have just started to brown around the edges. Remove and set aside.

3. Assemble tacos by layering a few spoonfuls of salsa on a tortilla, then layer with black beans, roasted veggies, and desired toppings. Serve warm.

26. Vegetarian Moo Shu

Prep Time: 20 Minutes

Cook Time: 30 Minutes

Servings: 8

Ingredients

Moo Shu Ingredients:

- 1 batch crispy tofu (see below)
- 1 batch sauce (see below)
- 2 tablespoons peanut oil (or olive oil)
- 2 large eggs, whisked
- 8 ounces shiitake mushrooms, stemmed and thinly sliced
- 4 cloves garlic, minced or pressed
- 1 (14-ounce) bag coleslaw
- 1/2 cup thinly-sliced green onions
- For serving: flour tortillas, lettuce cups, rice or quinoa
- Toppings: hoisin sauce, extra green onions, toasted sesame seeds

Crispy Tofu Ingredients:

- 14 ounces extra-firm tofu

- 2 teaspoons cornstarch

- 1 teaspoon fine sea salt

- 1/2 teaspoon black pepper

- 1 tablespoon peanut oil (or olive oil)

Sauce Ingredients:

- 1/2 cup hoisin sauce

- 1/4 cup rice vinegar

- 2 tablespoons oyster sauce

- 2 tablespoons low-sodium soy sauce

- 1 teaspoon toasted sesame oil

- 1/4 teaspoon freshly-cracked black pepper

Instructions

To Make The Moo Shu:

1. Prepare the crispy tofu (if using) and sauce. See instructions below.

2. Meanwhile, heat 1 tablespoon oil in a large non-stick sauté pan over medium heat. Add the whisked eggs and let then cooked undisturbed for 2-3 minutes until they are mostly set and form an omelet. Flip the omelet and cook for 1 more minute on the second side. Then

transfer the omelet to a separate cutting board, and roughly chop it into small, thin pieces. Set aside.

3. Return the pan to the stove, and increase heat to high heat. Add 1 more tablespoon of oil and heat until shimmering. Then add the mushrooms and sauté for 3-4 minutes, stirring occasionally, until cooked and lightly browned. Add the coleslaw and half of the scallions. Saute for 2-3 minutes more, or until the cabbage has softened to your liking.

4. Add in the cooked tofu, 2/3 of the sauce, half of the green onions. Toss until combined.

5. Taste and season with additional salt and pepper if needed.

6. Serve over flour tortillas, lettuce cups, rice, or quinoa. Drizzle with the remaining sauce, and sprinkle with your desired garnishes. Then serve warm and enjoy!

To Make The Crispy Tofu:

1. Slice your block of tofu into 1/4-inch-thick slabs. Lay some paper towels or a clean tea towel on a large flat surface, like a cutting board, and lay the slabs in a single layer on top of the paper towels. Cover with another layer of paper towels. Then place a second cutting board on top of the tofu, and stack a bunch of heavy cans or pots or whatever you can safely balance

on top of the cutting board. The idea is to put a lot of pressure/weight on the tofu, which will help the excess water to press out into the paper towels. Let the tofu drain for at least 15-30 minutes.

2. Once the tofu is ready to go, slice it into your desired shapes. (I made thin strips, which you can see in the photos above.) Add the tofu to a large mixing bowl, sprinkle it evenly with the cornstarch, salt and pepper. Then toss until the tofu is evenly coated in the cornstarch mixture.

3. Heat oil in a large non-stick sauté pan over medium-high heat. Add the tofu and arrange it in a single layer. (You may need to do this in two batches if your pan isn't large enough for the tofu to all fit in a single layer.) Cook the tofu undisturbed until it is browned on the bottom side, about 2 minutes. Flip the tofu and cook until the second side is browned, about 1-2 minutes. Give the whole mixture a gentle toss and cook for 1 minuter, stirring occasionally, until the tofu is browned to your liking.

4. Transfer the tofu to a clean plate and set aside until ready to use.

To Make The Sauce:

1. Whisk all ingredients together in a small bowl until combined.

27. Roasted Cauliflower Orzo Salad

Prep Time: 15 Minutes

Cook Time: 25 Minutes

Servings: 10

Ingredients

Roasted Cauliflower Orzo Salad Ingredients:

- 12 ounces uncooked pasta (I used orzo)
- 2 large handfuls fresh baby arugula
- 1 batch roasted cauliflower (see below)
- 1 cup Kalamata olives, pitted and halved
- 2/3 cup roughy-chopped sun-dried tomatoes
- 1/2 cup crumbled feta or goat cheese
- 1/2 cup toasted pine nuts
- Half a small red onion, thinly sliced
- 1 batch lemon vinaigrette

Roasted Cauliflower Ingredients:

- 1 head cauliflower
- 1 tablespoon olive oil
- Kosher salt and freshly-cracked black pepper

Lemon Vinaigrette Ingredients:

- 1/4 cup olive oil
- 3 tablespoons freshly-squeezed lemon juice
- 3 tablespoons finely-chopped fresh parsley leaves
- 2 tablespoons red wine vinegar
- 1/2 teaspoon kosher salt
- 1/4 teaspoon freshly-cracked black pepper

Instructions

To Make The Roasted Cauliflower Orzo Salad:

2. Cook the pasta in a large stockpot of generously-salted water until it is al dente, according to package directions. Drain pasta and rinse under cold water for about 20-30 seconds until no longer hot. Set aside.
3. In a large mixing bowl, combine the cooked pasta, roasted cauliflower, olives, sun-dried tomatoes, crumbled cheese, pine nuts, red onion, and vinaigrette. Toss until evenly combined.
4. Serve immediately, or cover and refrigerate for up to 3 days.

To Make The Roasted Cauliflower:

1. Heat oven to 400°F.
2. Add the cauliflower to a large mixing bowl, drizzle evenly with olive oil, and toss until combined. (You can also do this directly on the baking sheet.) Turn the cauliflower out onto a large baking sheet, and spread out in a single layer. Season evenly with a few generous pinches of salt and pepper.
3. Bake uncovered for about 25-30 minutes, or until the cauliflower is lightly browned and tender. Remove from the oven, and set aside until ready to use.

To Make The Lemon Vinaigrette:

1. Whisk all ingredients together in a small bowl (or shake in a mason jar) until completely combined.

28. Italian Sausage, Kale & Orzo Stuffed Tomatoes

Prep Time: 5 Minutes

Cook Time: 15 Minutes

Servings: 6

Ingredients

- 8 oz. (half pound) Italian sausage
- 1 cup diced white onion
- 2 cloves garlic, minced
- 2 cups chopped kale
- 1/2 cup chicken broth
- 1/2 cup heavy cream or half and half
- 8 oz. orzo
- 4–6 large tomatoes, cored and hollowed out
- 1/2 cup toasted pine nuts (for garnish)
- 1/2 cup shredded Parmesan cheese (for garnish)

Instructions

2. Heat a large skillet over medium-high heat. Add Italian sausage and cook until browned, crumbling while it

cooks. Remove cooked sausage from pan with a slotted spoon.

3. Add the onion and garlic to the pan, and cook in the sausage grease for 5 minutes until the onion is cooked and translucent. Add the kale and chicken broth. Cover and cook for an additional 5 minutes until the kale is wilted and cooked. Reduce heat to low and add in the heavy cream (or half and half) and the cooked sausage. Stir to combine.

4. Meanwhile, cook the orzo in a large pot of boiling, generously-salted water according to package instructions. When cooked, use a slotted spoon to add the orzo plus a half cup of reserved pasta water to the sausage and kale mixture. Stir until combined, then remove from heat. Spoon the pasta into the hollowed-out tomatoes and garnish with toasted pine nuts and Parmesan cheese.

29. Hawaiian Bbq Chicken Bowls

Prep Time: 15 Minutes

Cook Time: 10 Minutes

Servings: 4

Ingredients

- 2 tablespoons olive oil, divided
- 1 pound boneless skinless chicken breasts, cut into bite-sized pieces
- Sea salt and freshly-cracked black pepper
- 2 bell peppers (I used one yellow, one red), cored and cut into bite-sized pieces
- 1 small red onion, peeled and cut into bite-sized pieces
- 1 small fresh pineapple, peeled, cored, and cut into bite-sized pieces
- 2/3 cup good-quality bbq sauce*, homemade or store-bought
- Optional toppings: lemon slices, finely-chopped fresh cilantro

Instructions

1. Heat 1 tablespoon oil in a large sauté pan over medium-high heat. Add chicken, season it with a few pinches of salt and pepper. Sauté for 4-5 minutes, stirring and flipping occasionally, until the chicken is cooked through and no longer pink inside. Transfer chicken to a clean plate, and set aside.

2. Add the remaining tablespoon of oil to the sauté pan. Add peppers and onion, and sauté for 3 minutes, stirring occasionally. Add the pineapple and sauté for 3-4 more minutes, stirring occasionally, until the vegetables reach your desired level of tenderness. (I like mine with a bit of crisp, not completely soft.)

3. Add the cooked chicken and bbq sauce to the sauté pan with the veggies, and toss everything until combined. Taste and season with additional salt and pepper as needed.

4. Serve immediately over rice or quinoa (or plain, or whatever sounds good), garnished with your desired toppings. Or, refrigerate in airtight containers for up to 3 days, or freeze for up to 3 months.

30. Peach Gazpacho

Prep Time: 10 Minutes

Cook Time: 00 Minutes

Servings: 6

Ingredients

- 1 pound peaches, pitted and roughly chopped
- 1 pound Roma tomatoes, cored and roughly chopped
- 1 slice whole wheat bread
- Half of an English cucumber (about 6 ounces), peeled and roughly chopped
- Half of a small red onion (about 2 ounces), peeled and roughly chopped
- ¼ cup packed fresh basil leaves (about 8 to 10 large leaves)
- 3 tablespoons olive oil
- 2 to 3 teaspoons sherry vinegar, to taste
- 1 teaspoon fine sea salt
- A few twists of freshly-ground black pepper
- 2 small cloves garlic

- Optional garnishes: chopped peaches, cucumber, fresh basil, hemp seeds, croutons, chopped nuts, and/or a drizzle of olive oil

Instructions

1. Blend. Combine all ingredients in a blender and purée until smooth.
2. Season. Taste and season with additional salt, pepper, sherry vinegar, and/or basil if needed.
3. Strain (optional). Strain the mixture through a large fine mesh strainer, if you would like a silky smooth texture.
4. Chill. Refrigerate in a sealed container for at least 3 to 4 hours, or until completely chilled.
5. Serve. Serve cold, topped with your desired garnishes.

www.ingramcontent.com/pod-product-compliance
Lightning Source LLC
Chambersburg PA
CBHW061004260726
48661CB00005B/2044